Text copyright © Pat Thomas 2003
Illustrations copyright © Lesley Harker 2003

Editor: Liz Gogerly
Concept design: Kate Buxton
Design: Jean Scott-Moncrieff

Published in Great Britain in 2003 by Hodder Wayland,
an imprint of Hodder Children's Books
This paperback edition published in 2004

British Library Cataloguing in Publication Data

Thomas, Pat, 1959-
   I can be safe : a first look at safety
   1.offenses against the person - Prevention -
   Juvenile literature 2.Accidents - Prevention
   - Juvenile literature
   I.Title II.Harker, Lesley
   613.6

   ISBN 0 7502 4265 5

Printed in China by WKT Company Limited

Hodder Children's Books
A division of Hodder Headline Limited
338 Euston Road
London NW1 3BH

I Can Be Safe

A FIRST LOOK AT SAFETY

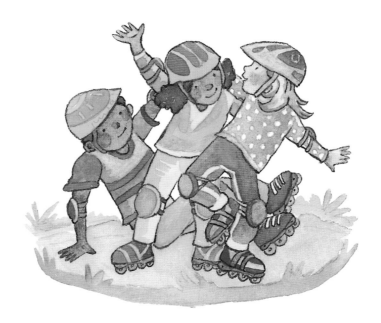

PAT THOMAS
ILLUSTRATED BY LESLEY HARKER

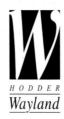

HODDER
Wayland

an imprint of Hodder Children's Books

Everyone needs to feel safe.

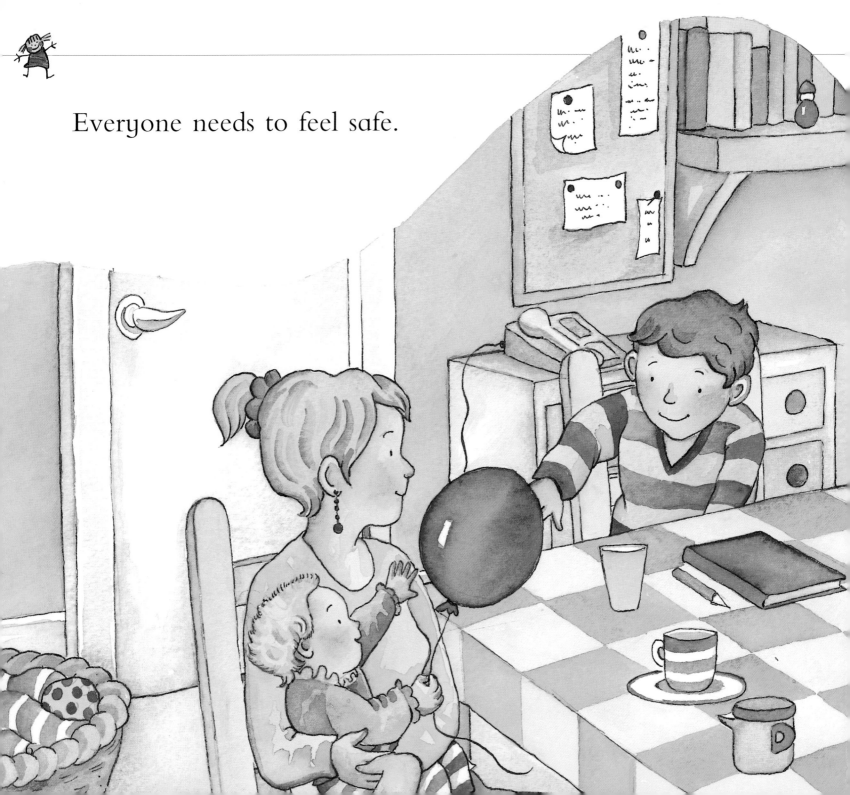

Most of us have special places we go and special people we know that make us feel safe.

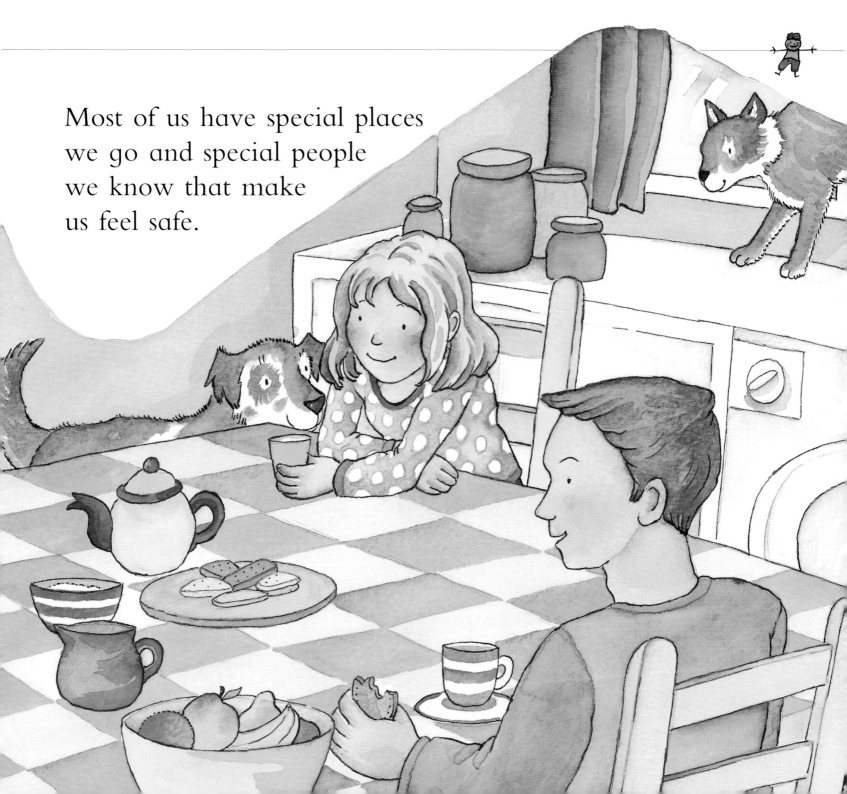

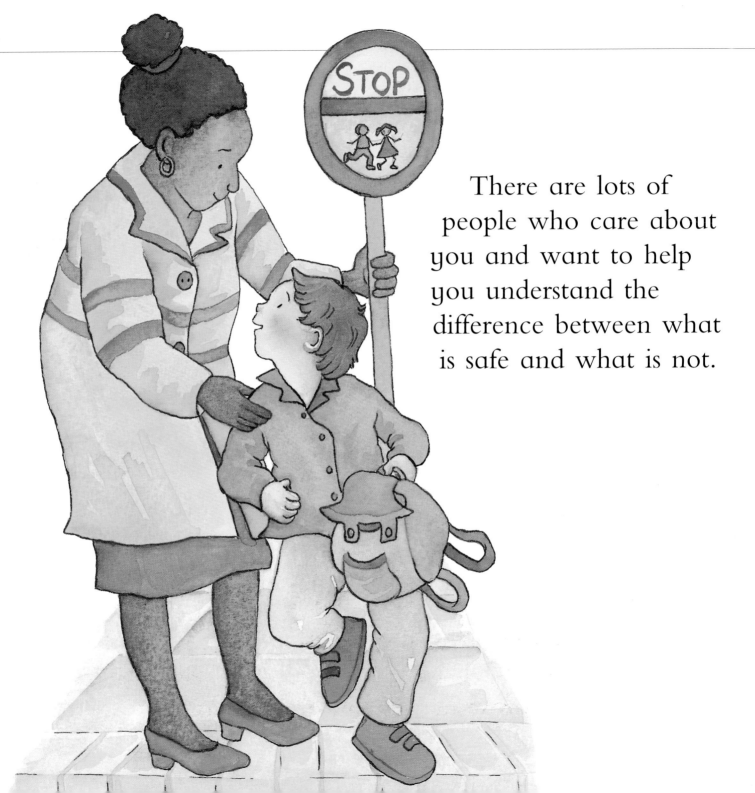

There are lots of
people who care about
you and want to help
you understand the
difference between what
is safe and what is not.

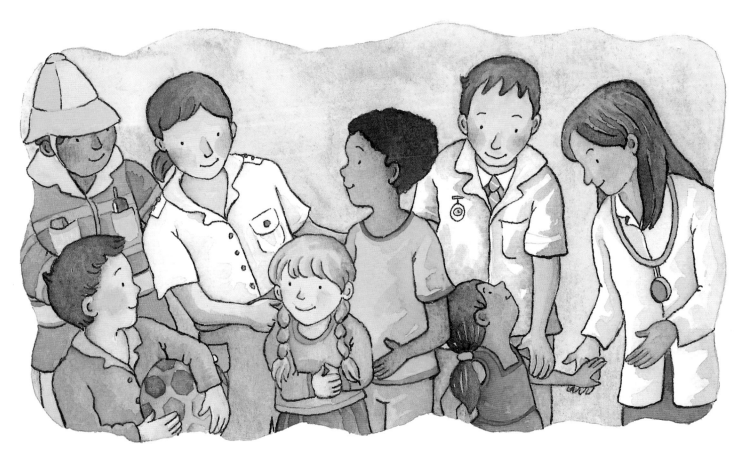

Your parents, teachers and other adults in your
community all want to help you learn all you
can about being safe so that you can
grow up healthy and strong.

You probably already know lots of different ways to keep yourself safe. Maybe you wear special clothing when you play sports.

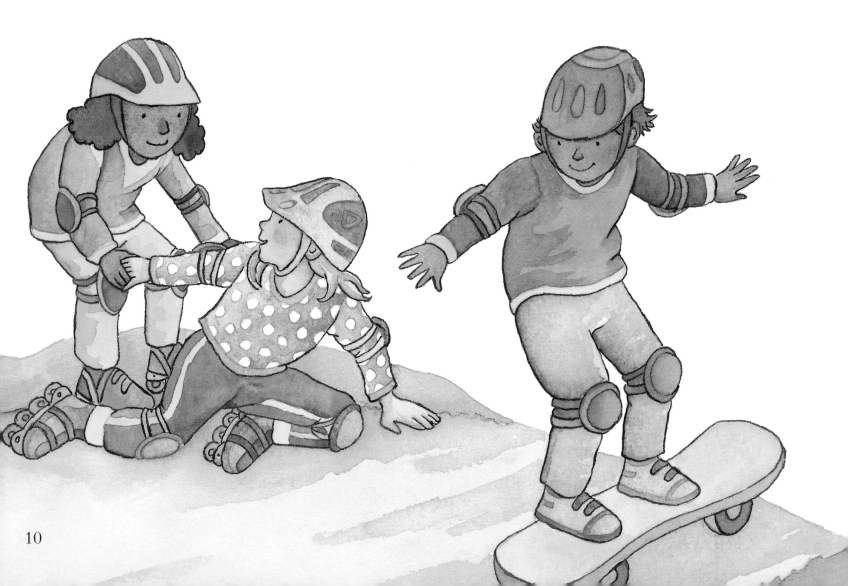

You may stop, look and listen before crossing a road. Or maybe you know to hold on to someone's hand in crowded places.

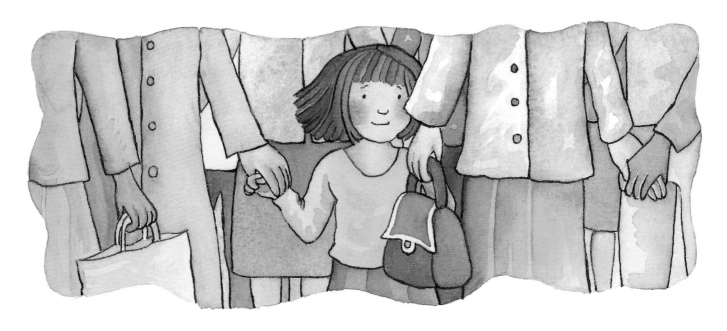

What about you?

What other things can you do to stay safe?
At home? At school?
In the playground? On the street?

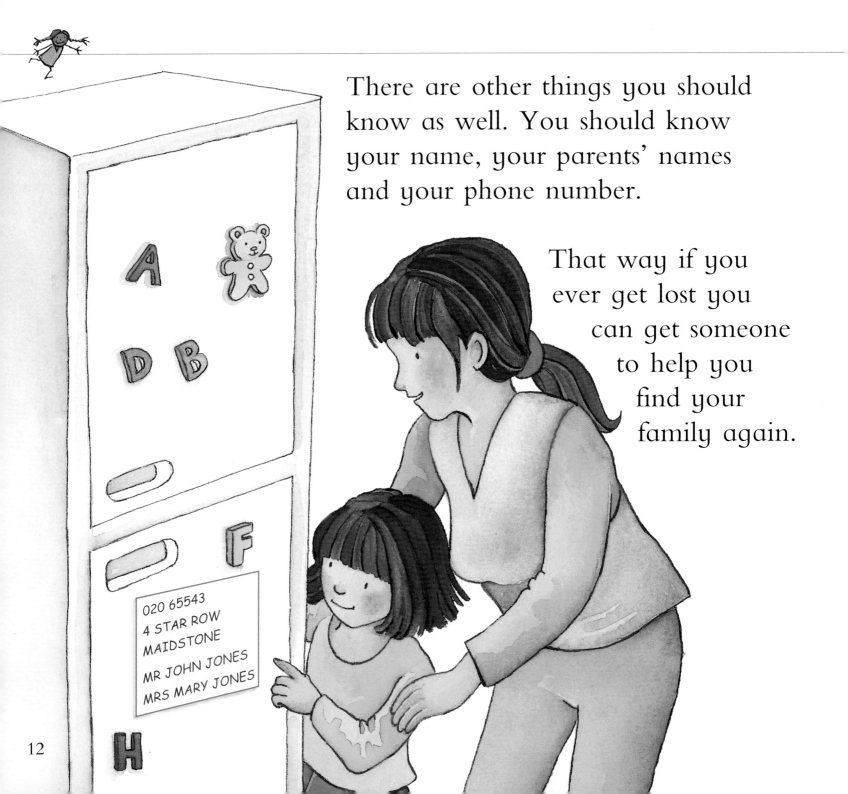

There are other things you should know as well. You should know your name, your parents' names and your phone number.

That way if you ever get lost you can get someone to help you find your family again.

020 65543
4 STAR ROW
MAIDSTONE

MR JOHN JONES
MRS MARY JONES

You should also know how to dial the emergency services in case of an accident.

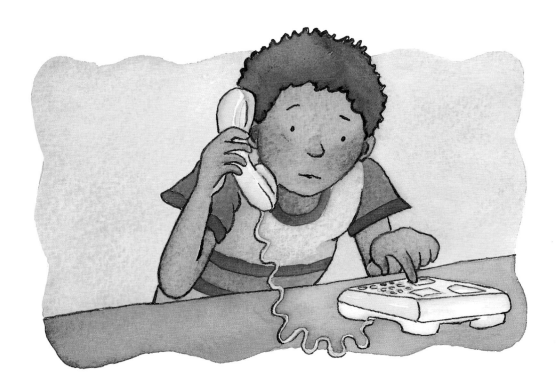

What about you?

Do you know this important information about yourself? Have you talked with your parents about what to do in emergencies? What have they said?

Did you know that each of us also has a special feeling that lets us know when things are not safe? This feeling is called instinct and it helps you know when something is wrong or you are in danger.

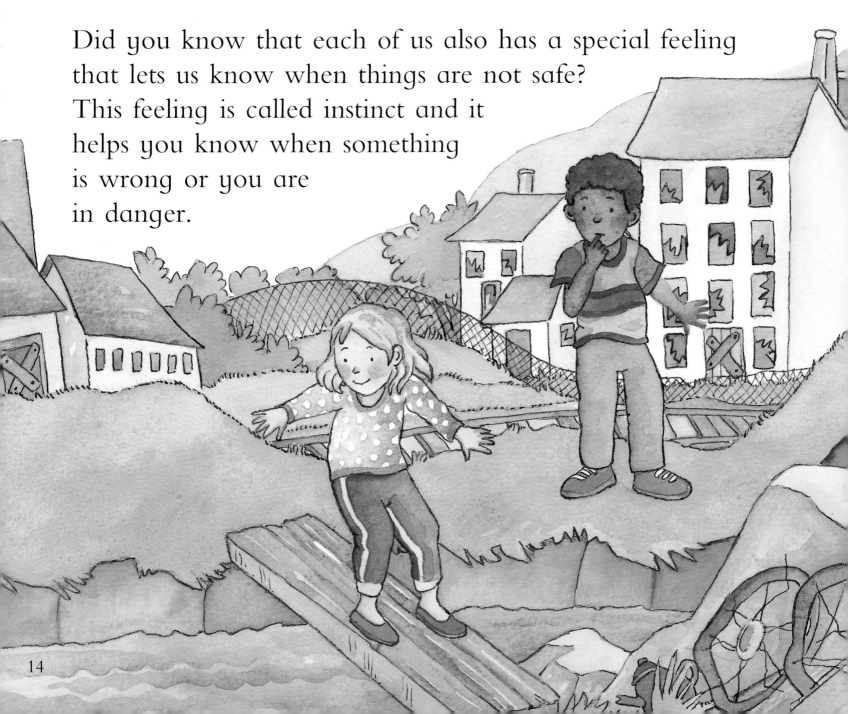

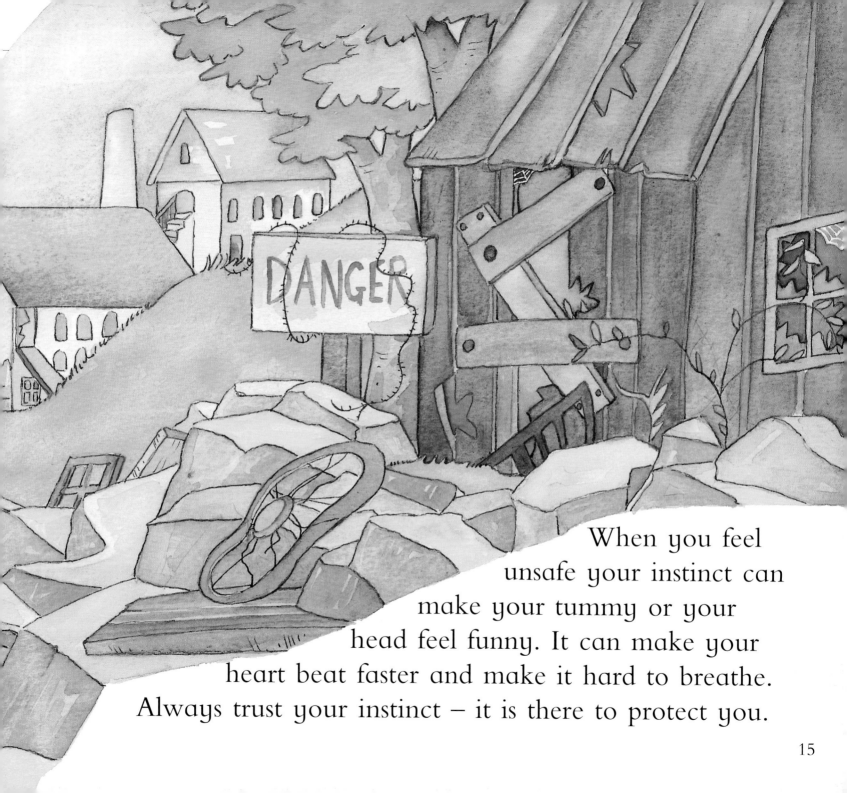

When you feel unsafe your instinct can make your tummy or your head feel funny. It can make your heart beat faster and make it hard to breathe. Always trust your instinct – it is there to protect you.

15

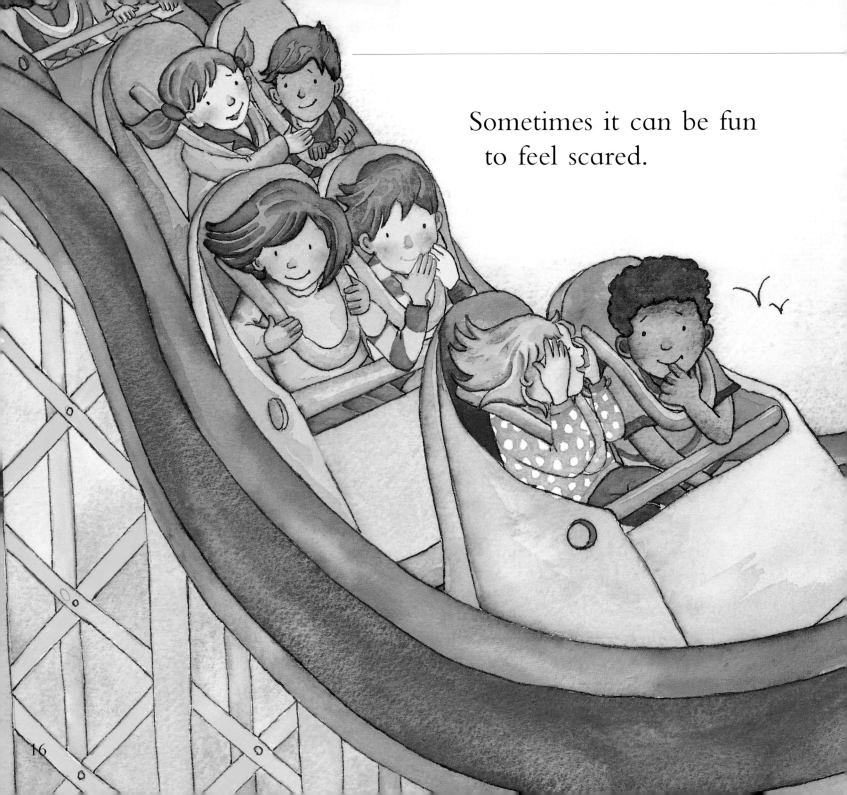

Sometimes it can be fun
to feel scared.

16

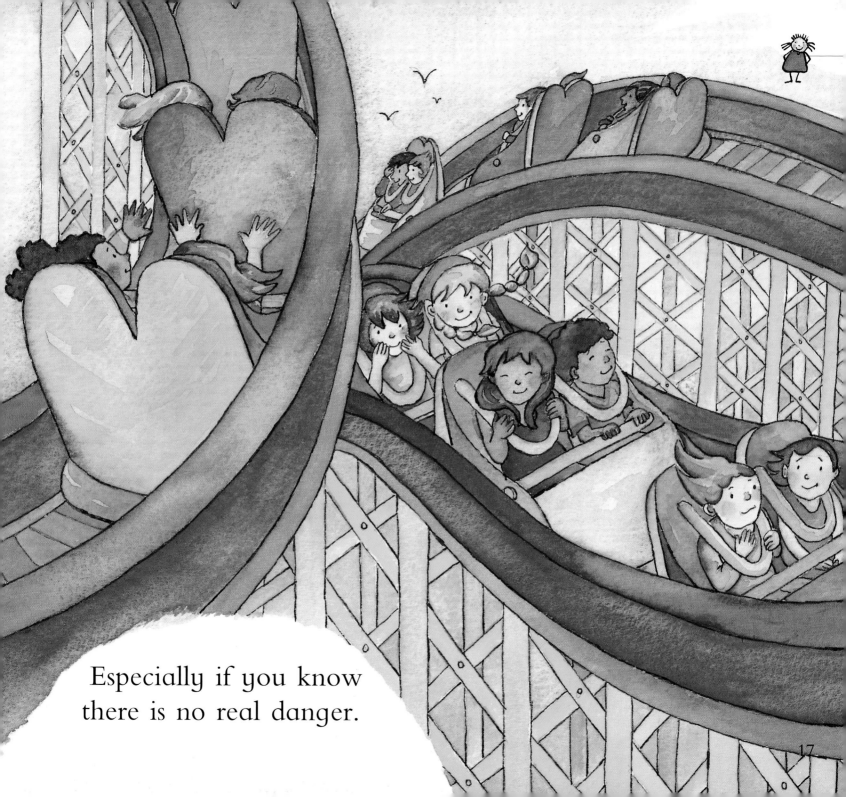

Especially if you know
there is no real danger.

But sometimes you feel scared for a good reason.

Like when someone you do not trust tries to talk to you or touch you.

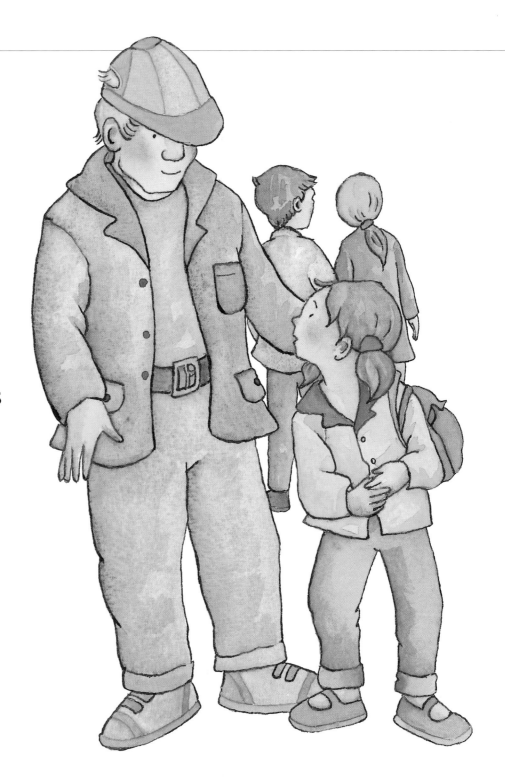

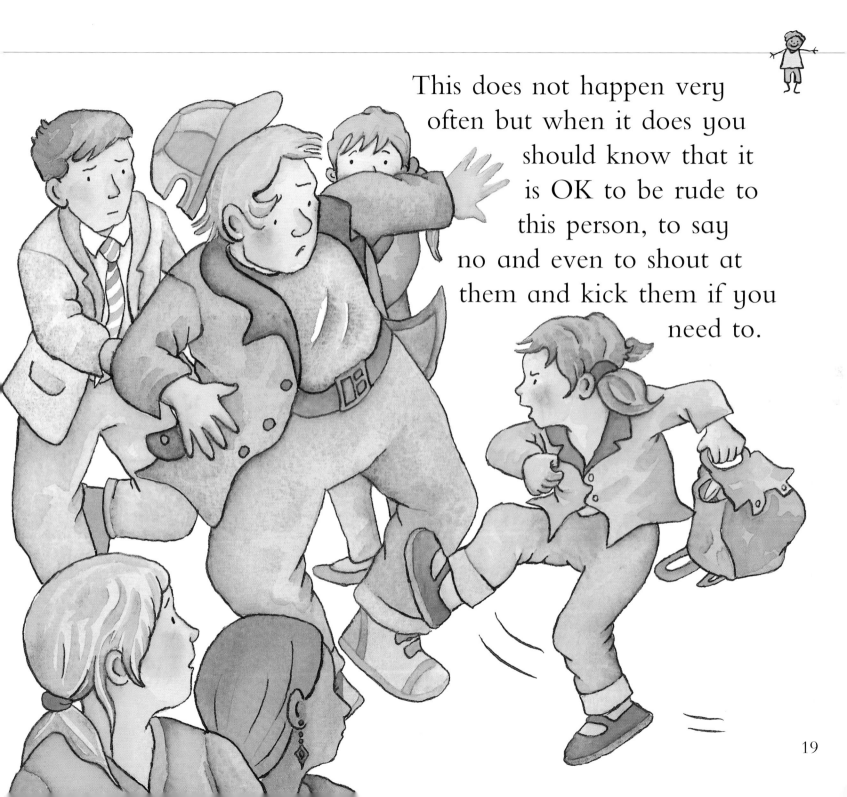

This does not happen very often but when it does you should know that it is OK to be rude to this person, to say no and even to shout at them and kick them if you need to.

19

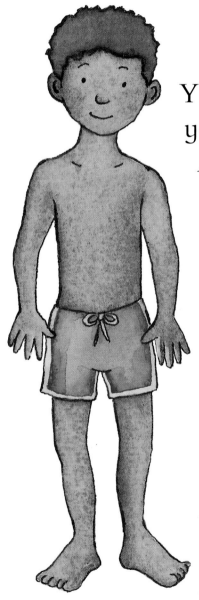

Your body belongs to you and you have a right to protect it. A good rule to remember is that people – especially those you don't feel comfortable with – should never touch any part of your body that is covered by your swimsuit.

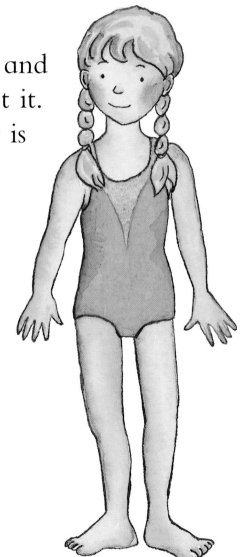

If this happens you should tell a parent or trusted grown-up. They can make sure it does not happen again.

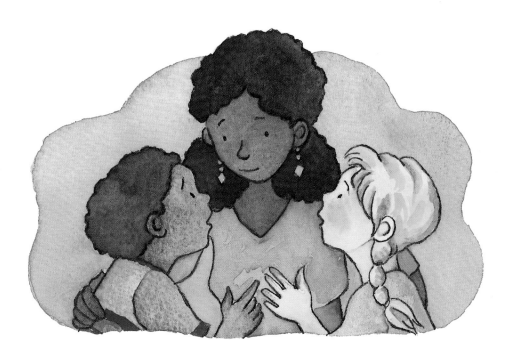

What about you?

Can you think of some other ways to stay safe if a stranger, or even someone you know but do not trust, gets too close to you? What do your parents say you should do?

Sometimes in order to be safe you have
to learn a new skill or a new set of rules.

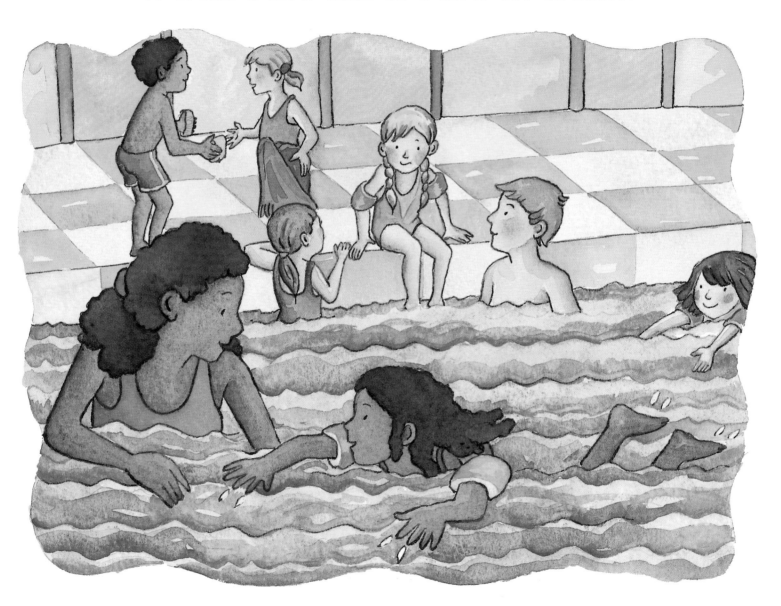

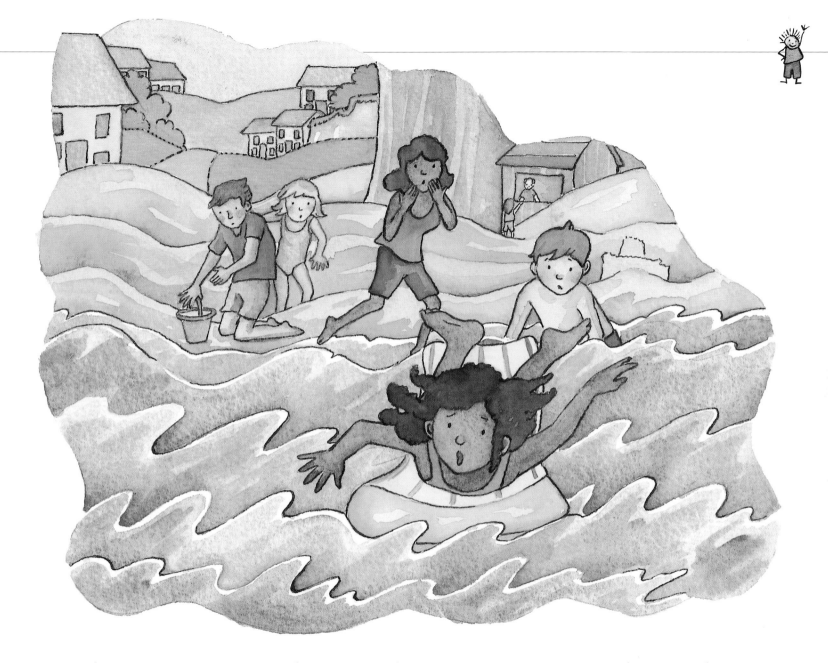

And sometimes you have to learn to say no to things that look fun but your feelings tell you could be dangerous.

Everyone forgets to act safely once in a while. We have all got lost or scared or hurt at sometime in our lives.

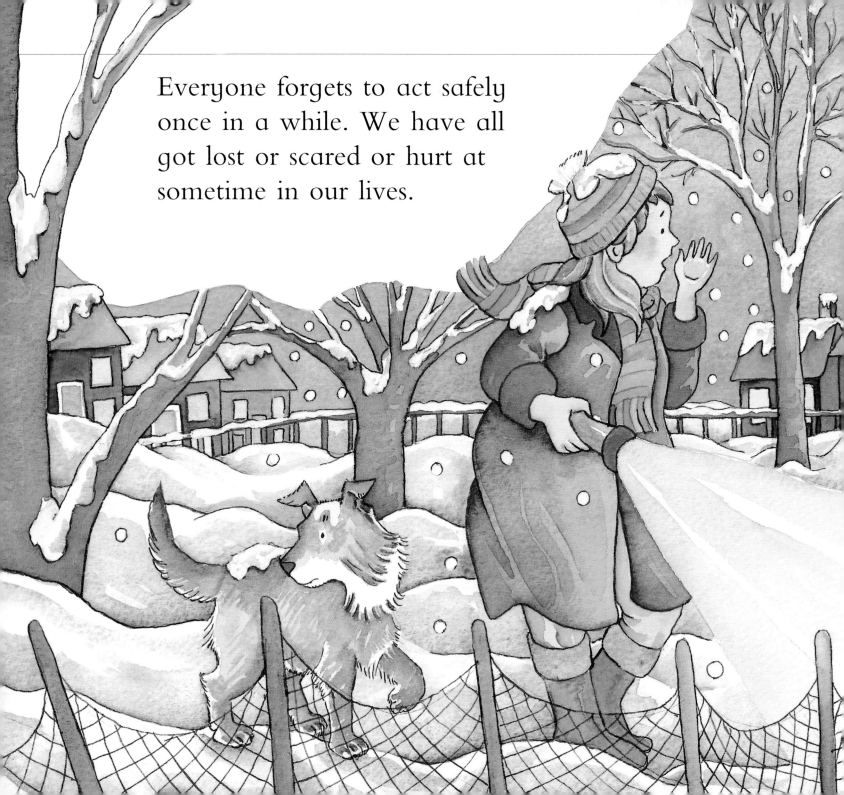

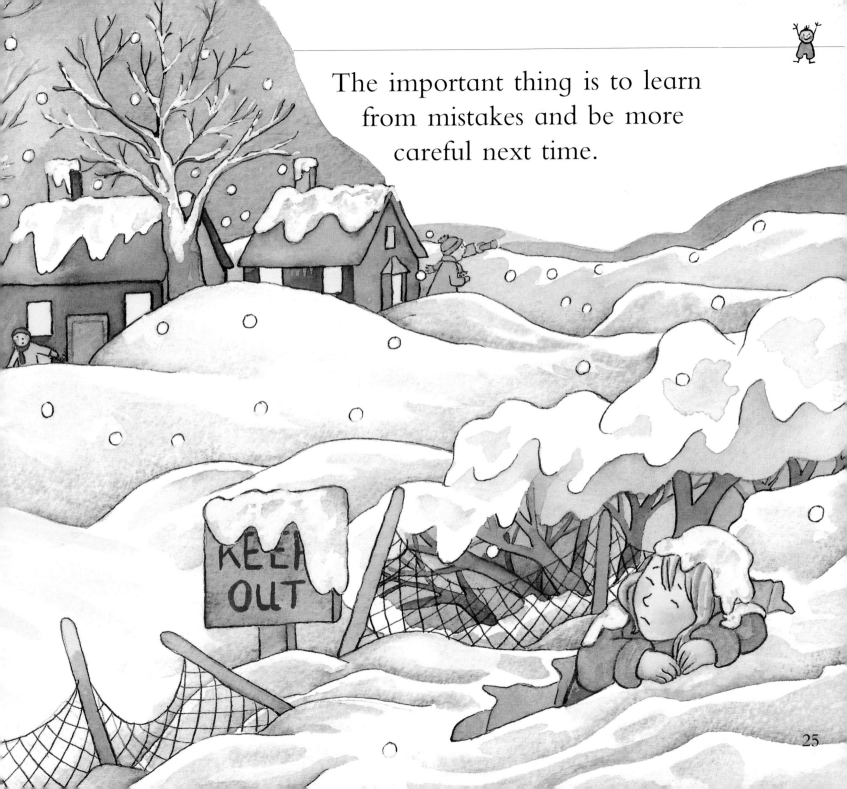

The important thing is to learn from mistakes and be more careful next time.

KEEP OUT

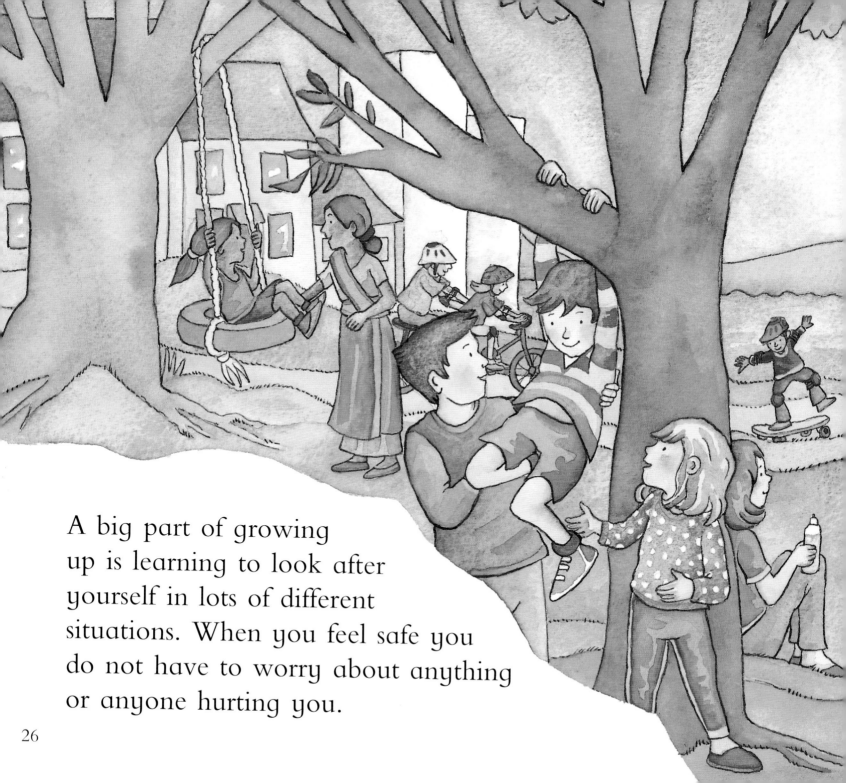

A big part of growing up is learning to look after yourself in lots of different situations. When you feel safe you do not have to worry about anything or anyone hurting you.

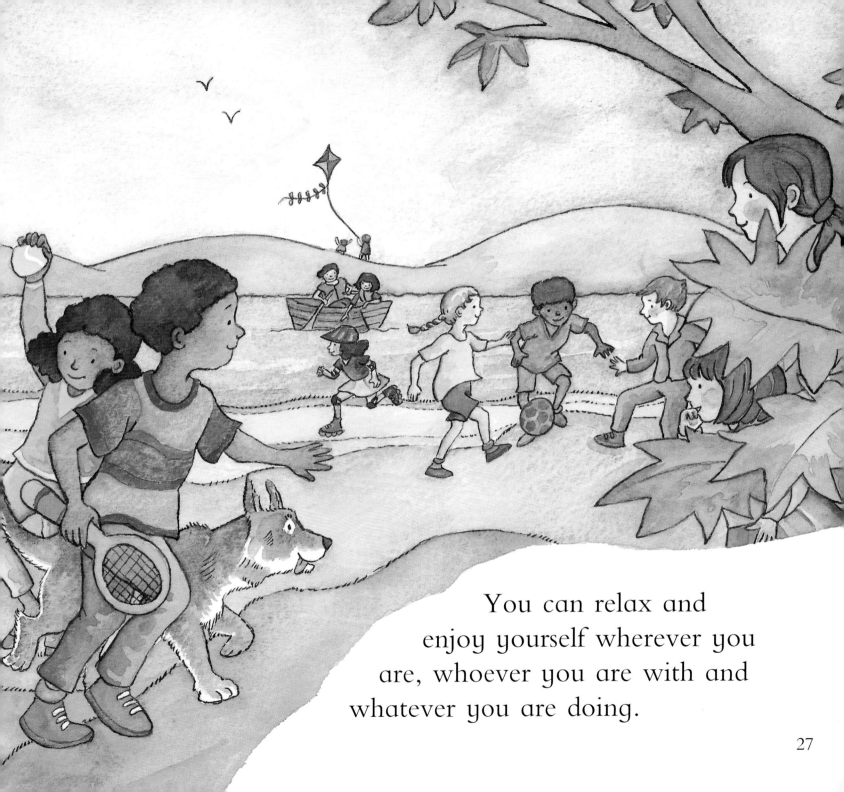

You can relax and
enjoy yourself wherever you
are, whoever you are with and
whatever you are doing.

HOW TO USE THIS BOOK

Keeping children safe is everyone's responsibility. Schools do an enormous amount of work in this area by providing lessons, talks and film and video presentations on many aspects of personal safety. Visits from police officers, fire fighters and others who are willing to talk about safety issues have become the norm. However lessons in safety must be continually reinforced by parents.

Consider some of the following suggestions for keeping your child safe in any situation:

First of all, keep your perspective. The majority of children do reach adulthood safe and well. Abductions and abuse, while devastating, are still rare.

Most parents provide day-to-day safety instructions without even thinking – 'Don't touch that it's hot', 'Hold my hand it's crowded in here', 'Look both ways before crossing the street', 'Wash your hands before you eat', 'Use your sunscreen'.

Bigger issues require a little more effort. As early as possible you should make a conscious effort to ensure your child knows their full name, their parents' full names, where they live (including the house number), street, city and postcode, and their full telephone number. In addition children should be given some instruction on dialling the emergency services for help.

Keep a list of important phone numbers somewhere obvious – for instance, stuck to the fridge with a colourful magnet – so that children can make use of these in an emergency. Making this kind of list could also be a good homework project for young children.

Be patient. Learning to take care of yourself is an ongoing lesson. Small children cannot possibly be expected to think through every situation from a safety point of view before acting. That's a parent's job. Just keep reinforcing the message and giving them opportunities to talk about it. Issuing orders is rarely a good way to get children to think about safety. Instead, lead by example. Learn to talk about safety issues as and when the opportunity arises – 'Did that boy look both ways before crossing the street?' 'Should that little girl be swimming on her own?' Let your child think it through and come up with the answers themselves.

Schools might consider holding a safety fair each year. Representatives of the police and fire departments, ambulance service, local sports and recreation facilities and local council could be invited to put up displays, give talks and give demonstrations. Follow up with classwork about what the children learned on the day.

You can talk to children about anything if you do it in a matter of fact way. Abuse and abduction, for example, can and should be talked about from an early age – just make sure the information you give is appropriate to your child's age and understanding of the world. Think through what you would like to say before you say it.

Reinforce the idea that a child's body is their personal property and that no one has the right to touch or hurt it. When discussing the topic of body privacy try to use real words such as 'penis' and 'vagina'. Let your child know that they must tell you if anyone ever talks about, teases them about, or tries to touch them in a way that feels wrong. Stress the fact that they should never keep any secrets from you concerning this subject, no matter what anyone tells them!

For a whole variety of reasons children may be left at home alone for varying lengths of time. Children need to understand that they must never let anyone know they are home alone. Nor should they answer the door when home alone unless a visitor is expected (and always check who is there before opening the door). If someone calls on the phone and asks to speak to an adult, a child at home alone should say that their parents are busy at the moment, take a message then politely hang up. Children should never give out any personal information (name, phone number, address, etc.) over the telephone or Internet.

To avoid a situation where a stranger tricks a child into coming with them, some families have a secret password that only the adults and children know. This password should only be used in an extreme emergency situation, for instance if a neighbour or someone they don't know has to unexpectedly pick up or take care of your child. Once the password is used, you need to change to a new password!

GLOSSARY

instinct when you just know something without being told. Your instinct is like your personal radar or x-ray vision. It helps you to see invisible clues that help you judge when something is right or not.

stranger someone you don't know. The most dangerous strangers are people you don't know who try to act like your friend. Or those who act one way in front of other adults but a different way when they are alone with you.

FURTHER READING

Look Out for Strangers
by Paul Humphreys and Alex Ramsay
(Evans Brothers, 2003)

Safety First
by Angela Royston (Heinemann Library, 2000)

The Berenstain Bears Learn About Strangers
by Stan Berenstain, Jan Berenstain
(Random House, 1985)

RESOURCES

NSPCC
Weston House
42 Curtain Road
London EC2A 3NH
020 7825 2500
Helpline: 0808 800 5000

Produces a range of publications about many aspects of child safety. Anyone can phone the free Childline helpline if they have questions about general issues in child safety or are fearful for a child's safety.

The Access Partnership
Hilton House
Lord Street
Stockport
SK1 3NA
0161 480 2323

A useful resource for parents and teachers focusing on key elements of personal, social and health education at all age levels. Lots of publications that can be bought by schools and parents and a website full of good links, games and quizzes for children.